THE ULTIMATE
blood sugar log book

A step-by-step guide to tracking blood sugar
and other common factors that affect blood sugar
to identify trends and live a healthier life with diabetes

CREATED BY KAYCEE PARKER

a type 1 diabetes warrior for 30+ years

www.DevotionsOnDiabetes.com

THE ULTIMATE BLOOD SUGAR LOG BOOK

www.DevotionsOnDiabetes.com

ISBN: 978-0-9991973-4-9 (paperback)

WELCOME
to the ultimate blood sugar log book

You are about to find out that this blood sugar log is different than others you may have seen or used in the past. The forms in this book are more comprehensive than many blood sugar logs.

That's because I know from my 30+ years with type 1 diabetes that managing diabetes well is about more than just glucose readings. It's about understanding the bigger picture of your health and how it impacts your diabetes. It's about looking at trends from the various factors that affect blood sugar. It's about gathering information and asking good questions to improve your health.

Yes, this log book is designed to help you track your blood sugar levels, but it will also help you track key lifestyle factors that can significantly influence them.

By paying attention to things like exercise, macronutrients, sleep quality, stress levels, and more, you can start to uncover patterns you may not otherwise see. Although this is not an exhaustive list of the things that impact blood sugar, here are several items you can track in this book:

Exercise plays an important role in insulin sensitivity and helping your body use insulin more effectively. Frequent physical activity, even light movement, can lower blood sugar levels and reduce the risk of long-term complications related to diabetes.

Counting macros gives insight into how different foods impact your blood sugar levels. Tracking the balance between carbs (fiber), fat, and protein can help you see trends and plan meals that result in a more stable blood sugar.

Post-meal blood sugar helps us see the fluctuations of our blood sugar after eating and taking medication. It can also help us with the proper timing of medications.

Sleep quality impacts more than just our mood. Poor sleep can increase insulin resistance and raise blood sugar levels. Tracking your rest can help you identify potential connections between sleep and blood sugar changes.

Stress (physical or emotional) can cause blood sugar spikes because of the release of cortisol, a hormone that increases glucose in the bloodstream. By tracking your stress levels, you can gain insight into how your mental state and emotions affect your blood sugar and your health overall.

Once you start tracking these values, you can start to see patterns and work with your doctor to make informed decisions for more stable and consistent blood sugar levels. And don't forget to celebrate progress as you go!

You may start to see trends develop as you track day to day. Another easy way to see trends is on the weekly summary pages. As you start to compare days side by side on this page each week, new insights may appear. This page also encourages you to celebrate goals you met and consider adjustments for the following week.

Do you have to track everything in this log book? No. You can certainly use whatever parts of it you want. And if this level of detail is overwhelming, start with what makes the most sense to you. You may be surprised what you find even if you're not utilizing this book to its fullest extent.

My goal in creating this book is to help you take a deep dive into several of the common factors that affect blood glucose. You can also share this information with your healthcare team. **Consult with your doctor before making any changes.**

This book was ultimately created to provide you with six weeks of intense tracking in order to look for trends and share with your healthcare team to help you manage diabetes better. And that can help empower you to make better choices and live a healthier life with diabetes!

Blessings,
Kaycee

PS. BE SURE TO CHECK OUT THE BONUS MATERIALS FOR YOU IN THE BACK OF THIS BOOK!

HOW TO USE
the ultimate blood sugar log book

First, you'll want to set your own personal goals on page 10 so you can celebrate your progress as you go. Then start tracking with week 1 day 1.

Below is an example of how to complete a daily worksheet. Fill in as much of it as you can in order to get the maximum benefit of this log book.

DAY ONE

date: March 17 (S) M T W T F S sleep hours: 7.5

fasting blood sugar: 117 time: 6:10 (am) pm

MORNING blood sugar: 136 time: 8:20 (am) pm

food/drink	calories	fat	carbs	fiber	protein
whole grain toast with 2 T. peanut butter	320	18	29	8	12
2 eggs	156	10	1	0	12
coffee with cream	40	3	1	0	0
totals:	516	31	31	8	24

medication: Humalog insulin dose: 3.6 units time: 8:30 (am) pm

post-meal blood sugar: 182 time: 10:30 (am) pm

SNACK blood sugar: 102 time: 2:30 am (pm)

food/drink	calories	fat	carbs	fiber	protein
2/3 c. greek yogurt with 1/4 c. granola	210	3	25	3	22

medication: Humalog insulin dose: 1.8 units time: 2:30 am (pm)

post-meal blood sugar: 139 time: 4:30 am (pm)

AVG B.S.	
138	

	calories	fat	carbs	fiber	protein
DAILY TOTALS	1,950	52	137	28	42

ENERGY LEVEL

1 2 3 4 5 6 (7) 8 9 10

LOW ———— HIGH

STRESS LEVEL

1 2 (3) 4 5 6 7 8 9 10

LOW ———— HIGH

EXERCISE

time	type	duration
2 pm	brisk walk outside	30 min

NOTES

Not active during the morning, needed more insulin.
Took correction at 10:30am.
Tired early in the evening.

There is ample room for notes throughout, so you can track other things like hormones, water intake, etc.

Once you have filled in details for each day of the week, it's time to look at the weekly summary sheet. This is another place we can get a good look at any patterns starting to emerge.

- By listing your blood sugars, you can see the range of numbers you have throughout the day, as well as when and how they fluctuate.
- By tracking your exercise, you can see if you met your activity goals and how that affects insulin sensitivity.
- By totaling your macros, you can see if you are in line with your nutrition goals.

If you need help with how to count carbs and other macros, you can get a step by step guide at: www.devotionsondiabetes.com/challenges-of-counting-carbs-for-diabetes/ or contact your healthcare team for personalized help.

If you need assistance with knowing the proper amount of macros for you personally each day, consult your diabetes dietitian or healthcare team.

There's something intentional and thoughtful about handwriting this information. It just makes you think. However, you may have access to data from a continuous glucose monitor and prefer not to track blood sugars manually here. That's perfectly fine. You can match up those reports against the rest of the data you track here to see the full picture. Feel free to use this journal however you believe it will be most beneficial to you!

MY PERSONAL GOALS

BLOOD SUGAR

The goal for my blood sugar in general is between: ______ – ______.

More specifically, my blood sugar goals are:

________ when I'm fasting ________ after meals

________ before meals ________ before bed

MACROS

My daily food and drink intake goals are: ________ calories ________ fiber

________ fat ________ protein

________ carbs

EXERCISE

My exercise goals are to complete:

________ minutes of cardio ________ times per week and

________ minutes of strength training ________ times per week.

SLEEP

My sleep goal is to consistently get ________ hours of sleep per night.

OTHER

Additional goals I have are: ____

____

____

WEEK ONE

DAY ONE

date: ____________ S M T W T F S sleep hours: ________

fasting blood sugar: ____________ time: ________ am pm

MORNING

blood sugar: ________ time: ________ am pm

food/drink	calories	fat	carbs	fiber	protein
totals:					

medication: ____________ dose: ________ time: ________ am pm

post-meal blood sugar: ________ time: ________ am pm

SNACK

blood sugar: ________ time: ________ am pm

food/drink	calories	fat	carbs	fiber	protein

medication: ____________ dose: ________ time: ________ am pm

post-meal blood sugar: ________ time: ________ am pm

MIDDAY

blood sugar: ________ time: ________ am pm

food/drink	calories	fat	carbs	fiber	protein
totals:					

medication: ____________ dose: ________ time: ________ am pm

post-meal blood sugar: ________ time: ________ am pm

SNACK

blood sugar: ________ time: ________ am pm

food/drink	calories	fat	carbs	fiber	protein

medication: ____________ dose: ________ time: ________ am pm

post-meal blood sugar: ________ time: ________ am pm

EVENING blood sugar: ____________ time: ____________ am pm

food/drink	calories	fat	carbs	fiber	protein
totals:					

medication: ______________________ dose: __________ time: __________ am pm

post-meal blood sugar: ____________ time: ____________ am pm

NIGHT blood sugar: ____________ time: ____________ am pm

food/drink	calories	fat	carbs	fiber	protein

medication: ______________________ dose: __________ time: __________ am pm

post-meal blood sugar: ____________ time: ____________ am pm

AVG B.S.	

	calories	fat	carbs	fiber	protein
DAILY TOTALS					

ENERGY LEVEL

1 2 3 4 5 6 7 8 9 10

LOW ———— HIGH

STRESS LEVEL

1 2 3 4 5 6 7 8 9 10

LOW ———— HIGH

EXERCISE

time	type	duration

NOTES

DAY TWO

date: ____________ S M T W T F S sleep hours: ________

fasting blood sugar: ____________ time: ________ am pm

MORNING

blood sugar: ________ time: ________ am pm

food/drink	calories	fat	carbs	fiber	protein
totals:					

medication: ____________ dose: ________ time: ________ am pm

post-meal blood sugar: ________ time: ________ am pm

SNACK

blood sugar: ________ time: ________ am pm

food/drink	calories	fat	carbs	fiber	protein

medication: ____________ dose: ________ time: ________ am pm

post-meal blood sugar: ________ time: ________ am pm

MIDDAY

blood sugar: ________ time: ________ am pm

food/drink	calories	fat	carbs	fiber	protein
totals:					

medication: ____________ dose: ________ time: ________ am pm

post-meal blood sugar: ________ time: ________ am pm

SNACK

blood sugar: ________ time: ________ am pm

food/drink	calories	fat	carbs	fiber	protein

medication: ____________ dose: ________ time: ________ am pm

post-meal blood sugar: ________ time: ________ am pm

EVENING blood sugar: ______________ time: ______________ am pm

food/drink	calories	fat	carbs	fiber	protein
totals:					

medication: ______________________________ dose: __________ time: __________ am pm

post-meal blood sugar: ______________ time: ______________ am pm

NIGHT blood sugar: ______________ time: ______________ am pm

food/drink	calories	fat	carbs	fiber	protein

medication: ______________________________ dose: __________ time: __________ am pm

post-meal blood sugar: ______________ time: ______________ am pm

AVG B.S.	

	calories	fat	carbs	fiber	protein
DAILY TOTALS					

ENERGY LEVEL

1 2 3 4 5 6 7 8 9 10

LOW ———————— HIGH

STRESS LEVEL

1 2 3 4 5 6 7 8 9 10

LOW ———————— HIGH

EXERCISE

time	type	duration

NOTES

DAY THREE

date: ______________ S M T W T F S sleep hours: __________

fasting blood sugar: ______________ time: __________ am pm

MORNING blood sugar: __________ time: __________ am pm

food/drink	calories	fat	carbs	fiber	protein
totals:					

medication: ____________________ dose: __________ time: __________ am pm

post-meal blood sugar: __________ time: __________ am pm

SNACK blood sugar: __________ time: __________ am pm

food/drink	calories	fat	carbs	fiber	protein

medication: ____________________ dose: __________ time: __________ am pm

post-meal blood sugar: __________ time: __________ am pm

MIDDAY blood sugar: __________ time: __________ am pm

food/drink	calories	fat	carbs	fiber	protein
totals:					

medication: ____________________ dose: __________ time: __________ am pm

post-meal blood sugar: __________ time: __________ am pm

SNACK blood sugar: __________ time: __________ am pm

food/drink	calories	fat	carbs	fiber	protein

medication: ____________________ dose: __________ time: __________ am pm

post-meal blood sugar: __________ time: __________ am pm

EVENING blood sugar: ________ time: ________ am pm

food/drink	calories	fat	carbs	fiber	protein
totals:					

medication: ________ dose: ________ time: ________ am pm

post-meal blood sugar: ________ time: ________ am pm

NIGHT blood sugar: ________ time: ________ am pm

food/drink	calories	fat	carbs	fiber	protein

medication: ________ dose: ________ time: ________ am pm

post-meal blood sugar: ________ time: ________ am pm

AVG B.S. ________

	calories	fat	carbs	fiber	protein
DAILY TOTALS					

ENERGY LEVEL

1 2 3 4 5 6 7 8 9 10

LOW —— HIGH

STRESS LEVEL

1 2 3 4 5 6 7 8 9 10

LOW —— HIGH

EXERCISE

time	type	duration

NOTES

DAY FOUR

date: ____________ S M T W T F S sleep hours: ________

fasting blood sugar: ____________ time: ________ am pm

MORNING

blood sugar: ________ time: ________ am pm

food/drink	calories	fat	carbs	fiber	protein
totals:					

medication: ____________ dose: ________ time: ________ am pm

post-meal blood sugar: ________ time: ________ am pm

SNACK

blood sugar: ________ time: ________ am pm

food/drink	calories	fat	carbs	fiber	protein

medication: ____________ dose: ________ time: ________ am pm

post-meal blood sugar: ________ time: ________ am pm

MIDDAY

blood sugar: ________ time: ________ am pm

food/drink	calories	fat	carbs	fiber	protein
totals:					

medication: ____________ dose: ________ time: ________ am pm

post-meal blood sugar: ________ time: ________ am pm

SNACK

blood sugar: ________ time: ________ am pm

food/drink	calories	fat	carbs	fiber	protein

medication: ____________ dose: ________ time: ________ am pm

post-meal blood sugar: ________ time: ________ am pm

EVENING	blood sugar: ______		time: ______ am pm		
food/drink	calories	fat	carbs	fiber	protein
totals:					

medication: ______ dose: ______ time: ______ am pm

post-meal blood sugar: ______ time: ______ am pm

NIGHT	blood sugar: ______		time: ______ am pm		
food/drink	calories	fat	carbs	fiber	protein

medication: ______ dose: ______ time: ______ am pm

post-meal blood sugar: ______ time: ______ am pm

AVG B.S.	

	calories	fat	carbs	fiber	protein
DAILY TOTALS					

ENERGY LEVEL

1 2 3 4 5 6 7 8 9 10

LOW —— HIGH

STRESS LEVEL

1 2 3 4 5 6 7 8 9 10

LOW —— HIGH

EXERCISE

time	type	duration

NOTES

DAY FIVE

date: ____________ S M T W T F S sleep hours: ________

fasting blood sugar: ____________ time: ________ am pm

MORNING blood sugar: ________ time: ________ am pm

food/drink	calories	fat	carbs	fiber	protein
totals:					

medication: ________________ dose: ________ time: ________ am pm

post-meal blood sugar: ________ time: ________ am pm

SNACK blood sugar: ________ time: ________ am pm

food/drink	calories	fat	carbs	fiber	protein

medication: ________________ dose: ________ time: ________ am pm

post-meal blood sugar: ________ time: ________ am pm

MIDDAY blood sugar: ________ time: ________ am pm

food/drink	calories	fat	carbs	fiber	protein
totals:					

medication: ________________ dose: ________ time: ________ am pm

post-meal blood sugar: ________ time: ________ am pm

SNACK blood sugar: ________ time: ________ am pm

food/drink	calories	fat	carbs	fiber	protein

medication: ________________ dose: ________ time: ________ am pm

post-meal blood sugar: ________ time: ________ am pm

EVENING

blood sugar: ____________ time: ____________ am pm

food/drink	calories	fat	carbs	fiber	protein
totals:					

medication: ______________________ dose: __________ time: __________ am pm

post-meal blood sugar: ____________ time: ____________ am pm

NIGHT

blood sugar: ____________ time: ____________ am pm

food/drink	calories	fat	carbs	fiber	protein

medication: ______________________ dose: __________ time: __________ am pm

post-meal blood sugar: ____________ time: ____________ am pm

AVG B.S.	

	calories	fat	carbs	fiber	protein
DAILY TOTALS					

ENERGY LEVEL

1 2 3 4 5 6 7 8 9 10

LOW ———————— HIGH

STRESS LEVEL

1 2 3 4 5 6 7 8 9 10

LOW ———————— HIGH

EXERCISE

time	type	duration

NOTES

DAY SIX

date: ____________ S M T W T F S sleep hours: ________

fasting blood sugar: ____________ time: ________ am pm

MORNING

blood sugar: ________ time: ________ am pm

food/drink	calories	fat	carbs	fiber	protein
totals:					

medication: ________________ dose: ________ time: ________ am pm

post-meal blood sugar: ________ time: ________ am pm

SNACK

blood sugar: ________ time: ________ am pm

food/drink	calories	fat	carbs	fiber	protein

medication: ________________ dose: ________ time: ________ am pm

post-meal blood sugar: ________ time: ________ am pm

MIDDAY

blood sugar: ________ time: ________ am pm

food/drink	calories	fat	carbs	fiber	protein
totals:					

medication: ________________ dose: ________ time: ________ am pm

post-meal blood sugar: ________ time: ________ am pm

SNACK

blood sugar: ________ time: ________ am pm

food/drink	calories	fat	carbs	fiber	protein

medication: ________________ dose: ________ time: ________ am pm

post-meal blood sugar: ________ time: ________ am pm

EVENING blood sugar: ____________ time: ____________ am pm

food/drink	calories	fat	carbs	fiber	protein
totals:					

medication: ____________ dose: ____________ time: ____________ am pm

post-meal blood sugar: ____________ time: ____________ am pm

NIGHT blood sugar: ____________ time: ____________ am pm

food/drink	calories	fat	carbs	fiber	protein

medication: ____________ dose: ____________ time: ____________ am pm

post-meal blood sugar: ____________ time: ____________ am pm

AVG B.S.	

	calories	fat	carbs	fiber	protein
DAILY TOTALS					

ENERGY LEVEL

1 2 3 4 5 6 7 8 9 10

LOW ——— HIGH

STRESS LEVEL

1 2 3 4 5 6 7 8 9 10

LOW ——— HIGH

EXERCISE

time	type	duration

NOTES

DAY SEVEN

date: ____________________ S M T W T F S sleep hours: __________

fasting blood sugar: ________________ time: ____________ am pm

MORNING

blood sugar: ____________ time: ____________ am pm

food/drink	calories	fat	carbs	fiber	protein
totals:					

medication: ____________________________ dose: __________ time: _________ am pm

post-meal blood sugar: ____________ time: ____________ am pm

SNACK

blood sugar: ____________ time: ____________ am pm

food/drink	calories	fat	carbs	fiber	protein

medication: ____________________________ dose: __________ time: _________ am pm

post-meal blood sugar: ____________ time: ____________ am pm

MIDDAY

blood sugar: ____________ time: ____________ am pm

food/drink	calories	fat	carbs	fiber	protein
totals:					

medication: ____________________________ dose: __________ time: _________ am pm

post-meal blood sugar: ____________ time: ____________ am pm

SNACK

blood sugar: ____________ time: ____________ am pm

food/drink	calories	fat	carbs	fiber	protein

medication: ____________________________ dose: __________ time: _________ am pm

post-meal blood sugar: ____________ time: ____________ am pm

EVENING blood sugar: ______ time: ______ am pm

food/drink	calories	fat	carbs	fiber	protein
totals:					

medication: ______ dose: ______ time: ______ am pm

post-meal blood sugar: ______ time: ______ am pm

NIGHT blood sugar: ______ time: ______ am pm

food/drink	calories	fat	carbs	fiber	protein

medication: ______ dose: ______ time: ______ am pm

post-meal blood sugar: ______ time: ______ am pm

AVG B.S.	

	calories	fat	carbs	fiber	protein
DAILY TOTALS					

ENERGY LEVEL

1 2 3 4 5 6 7 8 9 10

LOW ——— HIGH

STRESS LEVEL

1 2 3 4 5 6 7 8 9 10

LOW ——— HIGH

EXERCISE

time	type	duration

NOTES

WEEK ONE

WEEKLY SUMMARY

BLOOD SUGAR

	MORNING		SNACK		MIDDAY		SNACK		EVENING		NIGHT	
day	pre	post	pre	post	pre	post	pre	post	pre	post	pre	post
1												
2												
3												
4												
5												
6												
7												
AVG.												

MACROS

day	calories	fat	carbs	fiber	protein
1					
2					
3					
4					
5					
6					
7					
AVG.					

NOTES

ENERGY LEVEL AVERAGE

1 2 3 4 5 6 7 8 9 10

LOW —— HIGH

STRESS LEVEL AVERAGE

1 2 3 4 5 6 7 8 9 10

LOW —— HIGH

DAYS OF EXERCISE

1 2 3 4 5 6 7

AVG. MIN.

______

GOALS MET

ADJUSTMENTS

WEEK TWO

DAY ONE

date: ______________________ S M T W T F S sleep hours: ___________

fasting blood sugar: __________________ time: _____________ am pm

MORNING blood sugar: ______________ time: _____________ am pm

food/drink	calories	fat	carbs	fiber	protein
totals:					

medication: ______________________________ dose: ___________ time: __________ am pm

post-meal blood sugar: _____________ time: _____________ am pm

SNACK blood sugar: ______________ time: _____________ am pm

food/drink	calories	fat	carbs	fiber	protein

medication: ______________________________ dose: ___________ time: __________ am pm

post-meal blood sugar: _____________ time: _____________ am pm

MIDDAY blood sugar: ______________ time: _____________ am pm

food/drink	calories	fat	carbs	fiber	protein
totals:					

medication: ______________________________ dose: ___________ time: __________ am pm

post-meal blood sugar: _____________ time: _____________ am pm

SNACK blood sugar: ______________ time: _____________ am pm

food/drink	calories	fat	carbs	fiber	protein

medication: ______________________________ dose: ___________ time: __________ am pm

post-meal blood sugar: _____________ time: _____________ am pm

EVEVING	blood sugar: ______	time: ______ am pm			
food/drink	calories	fat	carbs	fiber	protein
totals:					

medication: ______ dose: ______ time: ______ am pm

post-meal blood sugar: ______ time: ______ am pm

NIGHT	blood sugar: ______	time: ______ am pm			
food/drink	calories	fat	carbs	fiber	protein

medication: ______ dose: ______ time: ______ am pm

post-meal blood sugar: ______ time: ______ am pm

AVG B.S.	

	calories	fat	carbs	fiber	protein
DAILY TOTALS					

ENERGY LEVEL

1 2 3 4 5 6 7 8 9 10

LOW —— HIGH

STRESS LEVEL

1 2 3 4 5 6 7 8 9 10

LOW —— HIGH

EXERCISE

time	type	duration

NOTES

DAY TWO

date: ____________ S M T W T F S sleep hours: ________

fasting blood sugar: ____________ time: ________ am pm

MORNING blood sugar: ________ time: ________ am pm

food/drink	calories	fat	carbs	fiber	protein
totals:					

medication: ____________ dose: ________ time: ________ am pm

post-meal blood sugar: ________ time: ________ am pm

SNACK blood sugar: ________ time: ________ am pm

food/drink	calories	fat	carbs	fiber	protein

medication: ____________ dose: ________ time: ________ am pm

post-meal blood sugar: ________ time: ________ am pm

MIDDAY blood sugar: ________ time: ________ am pm

food/drink	calories	fat	carbs	fiber	protein
totals:					

medication: ____________ dose: ________ time: ________ am pm

post-meal blood sugar: ________ time: ________ am pm

SNACK blood sugar: ________ time: ________ am pm

food/drink	calories	fat	carbs	fiber	protein

medication: ____________ dose: ________ time: ________ am pm

post-meal blood sugar: ________ time: ________ am pm

EVENING

blood sugar: ______________ time: ______________ am pm

food/drink	calories	fat	carbs	fiber	protein
totals:					

medication: ______________________________ dose: ___________ time: __________ am pm

post-meal blood sugar: ______________ time: ______________ am pm

NIGHT

blood sugar: ______________ time: ______________ am pm

food/drink	calories	fat	carbs	fiber	protein

medication: ______________________________ dose: ___________ time: __________ am pm

post-meal blood sugar: ______________ time: ______________ am pm

AVG B.S.	

	calories	fat	carbs	fiber	protein
DAILY TOTALS					

ENERGY LEVEL

1 2 3 4 5 6 7 8 9 10

LOW ———————— HIGH

STRESS LEVEL

1 2 3 4 5 6 7 8 9 10

LOW ———————— HIGH

EXERCISE

time	type	duration

NOTES

DAY THREE

date: ____________ S M T W T F S sleep hours: ________

fasting blood sugar: ____________ time: ________ am pm

MORNING blood sugar: ________ time: ________ am pm

food/drink	calories	fat	carbs	fiber	protein
totals:					

medication: ____________ dose: ________ time: ________ am pm

post-meal blood sugar: ________ time: ________ am pm

SNACK blood sugar: ________ time: ________ am pm

food/drink	calories	fat	carbs	fiber	protein

medication: ____________ dose: ________ time: ________ am pm

post-meal blood sugar: ________ time: ________ am pm

MIDDAY blood sugar: ________ time: ________ am pm

food/drink	calories	fat	carbs	fiber	protein
totals:					

medication: ____________ dose: ________ time: ________ am pm

post-meal blood sugar: ________ time: ________ am pm

SNACK blood sugar: ________ time: ________ am pm

food/drink	calories	fat	carbs	fiber	protein

medication: ____________ dose: ________ time: ________ am pm

post-meal blood sugar: ________ time: ________ am pm

EVENING blood sugar: ____________ time: ____________ am pm

food/drink	calories	fat	carbs	fiber	protein
totals:					

medication: ________________________ dose: __________ time: __________ am pm

post-meal blood sugar: ____________ time: ____________ am pm

NIGHT blood sugar: ____________ time: ____________ am pm

food/drink	calories	fat	carbs	fiber	protein

medication: ________________________ dose: __________ time: __________ am pm

post-meal blood sugar: ____________ time: ____________ am pm

AVG B.S.	

	calories	fat	carbs	fiber	protein
DAILY TOTALS					

ENERGY LEVEL

1 2 3 4 5 6 7 8 9 10

LOW ——— HIGH

STRESS LEVEL

1 2 3 4 5 6 7 8 9 10

LOW ——— HIGH

EXERCISE

time	type	duration

NOTES

DAY FOUR

date: ________ S M T W T F S sleep hours: ________

fasting blood sugar: ________ time: ________ am pm

MORNING

blood sugar: ________ time: ________ am pm

food/drink	calories	fat	carbs	fiber	protein
totals:					

medication: ________ dose: ________ time: ________ am pm

post-meal blood sugar: ________ time: ________ am pm

SNACK

blood sugar: ________ time: ________ am pm

food/drink	calories	fat	carbs	fiber	protein

medication: ________ dose: ________ time: ________ am pm

post-meal blood sugar: ________ time: ________ am pm

MIDDAY

blood sugar: ________ time: ________ am pm

food/drink	calories	fat	carbs	fiber	protein
totals:					

medication: ________ dose: ________ time: ________ am pm

post-meal blood sugar: ________ time: ________ am pm

SNACK

blood sugar: ________ time: ________ am pm

food/drink	calories	fat	carbs	fiber	protein

medication: ________ dose: ________ time: ________ am pm

post-meal blood sugar: ________ time: ________ am pm

EVENING blood sugar: ____________ time: ____________ am pm

food/drink	calories	fat	carbs	fiber	protein
totals:					

medication: ____________ dose: ____________ time: ____________ am pm

post-meal blood sugar: ____________ time: ____________ am pm

NIGHT blood sugar: ____________ time: ____________ am pm

food/drink	calories	fat	carbs	fiber	protein

medication: ____________ dose: ____________ time: ____________ am pm

post-meal blood sugar: ____________ time: ____________ am pm

AVG B.S.	

	calories	fat	carbs	fiber	protein
DAILY TOTALS					

ENERGY LEVEL

1 2 3 4 5 6 7 8 9 10

LOW ——— HIGH

STRESS LEVEL

1 2 3 4 5 6 7 8 9 10

LOW ——— HIGH

EXERCISE

time	type	duration

NOTES

DAY FIVE

date: ______________ S M T W T F S sleep hours: ________

fasting blood sugar: ______________ time: ________ am pm

MORNING

blood sugar: ________ time: ________ am pm

food/drink	calories	fat	carbs	fiber	protein
totals:					

medication: ______________ dose: ________ time: ________ am pm

post-meal blood sugar: ________ time: ________ am pm

SNACK

blood sugar: ________ time: ________ am pm

food/drink	calories	fat	carbs	fiber	protein

medication: ______________ dose: ________ time: ________ am pm

post-meal blood sugar: ________ time: ________ am pm

MIDDAY

blood sugar: ________ time: ________ am pm

food/drink	calories	fat	carbs	fiber	protein
totals:					

medication: ______________ dose: ________ time: ________ am pm

post-meal blood sugar: ________ time: ________ am pm

SNACK

blood sugar: ________ time: ________ am pm

food/drink	calories	fat	carbs	fiber	protein

medication: ______________ dose: ________ time: ________ am pm

post-meal blood sugar: ________ time: ________ am pm

EVENING

blood sugar: ____________ time: ____________ am pm

food/drink	calories	fat	carbs	fiber	protein
totals:					

medication: ____________________ dose: __________ time: __________ am pm

post-meal blood sugar: ____________ time: ____________ am pm

NIGHT

blood sugar: ____________ time: ____________ am pm

food/drink	calories	fat	carbs	fiber	protein

medication: ____________________ dose: __________ time: __________ am pm

post-meal blood sugar: ____________ time: ____________ am pm

AVG B.S.	

	calories	fat	carbs	fiber	protein
DAILY TOTALS					

ENERGY LEVEL

1 2 3 4 5 6 7 8 9 10

LOW ———————— HIGH

STRESS LEVEL

1 2 3 4 5 6 7 8 9 10

LOW ———————— HIGH

EXERCISE

time	type	duration

NOTES

DAY SIX

date: ____________ S M T W T F S sleep hours: ________

fasting blood sugar: ____________ time: ________ am pm

MORNING blood sugar: ________ time: ________ am pm

food/drink	calories	fat	carbs	fiber	protein
totals:					

medication: ____________ dose: ________ time: ________ am pm

post-meal blood sugar: ________ time: ________ am pm

SNACK blood sugar: ________ time: ________ am pm

food/drink	calories	fat	carbs	fiber	protein

medication: ____________ dose: ________ time: ________ am pm

post-meal blood sugar: ________ time: ________ am pm

MIDDAY blood sugar: ________ time: ________ am pm

food/drink	calories	fat	carbs	fiber	protein
totals:					

medication: ____________ dose: ________ time: ________ am pm

post-meal blood sugar: ________ time: ________ am pm

SNACK blood sugar: ________ time: ________ am pm

food/drink	calories	fat	carbs	fiber	protein

medication: ____________ dose: ________ time: ________ am pm

post-meal blood sugar: ________ time: ________ am pm

EVENING	blood sugar: ______	time: ______ am pm			
food/drink	calories	fat	carbs	fiber	protein
totals:					

medication: ______ dose: ______ time: ______ am pm

post-meal blood sugar: ______ time: ______ am pm

NIGHT	blood sugar: ______	time: ______ am pm			
food/drink	calories	fat	carbs	fiber	protein

medication: ______ dose: ______ time: ______ am pm

post-meal blood sugar: ______ time: ______ am pm

AVG B.S.	

	calories	fat	carbs	fiber	protein
DAILY TOTALS					

ENERGY LEVEL

1 2 3 4 5 6 7 8 9 10

LOW —— HIGH

STRESS LEVEL

1 2 3 4 5 6 7 8 9 10

LOW —— HIGH

EXERCISE

time	type	duration

NOTES

DAY SEVEN

date: ______________ S M T W T F S sleep hours: ________

fasting blood sugar: ______________ time: ________ am pm

MORNING blood sugar: ________ time: ________ am pm

food/drink	calories	fat	carbs	fiber	protein
totals:					

medication: ______________ dose: ________ time: ________ am pm

post-meal blood sugar: ________ time: ________ am pm

SNACK blood sugar: ________ time: ________ am pm

food/drink	calories	fat	carbs	fiber	protein

medication: ______________ dose: ________ time: ________ am pm

post-meal blood sugar: ________ time: ________ am pm

MIDDAY blood sugar: ________ time: ________ am pm

food/drink	calories	fat	carbs	fiber	protein
totals:					

medication: ______________ dose: ________ time: ________ am pm

post-meal blood sugar: ________ time: ________ am pm

SNACK blood sugar: ________ time: ________ am pm

food/drink	calories	fat	carbs	fiber	protein

medication: ______________ dose: ________ time: ________ am pm

post-meal blood sugar: ________ time: ________ am pm

EVENING blood sugar: ________ time: ________ am pm

food/drink	calories	fat	carbs	fiber	protein
totals:					

medication: ________ dose: ________ time: ________ am pm

post-meal blood sugar: ________ time: ________ am pm

NIGHT blood sugar: ________ time: ________ am pm

food/drink	calories	fat	carbs	fiber	protein

medication: ________ dose: ________ time: ________ am pm

post-meal blood sugar: ________ time: ________ am pm

AVG B.S. ________

	calories	fat	carbs	fiber	protein
DAILY TOTALS					

ENERGY LEVEL

1 2 3 4 5 6 7 8 9 10

LOW ———— HIGH

STRESS LEVEL

1 2 3 4 5 6 7 8 9 10

LOW ———— HIGH

EXERCISE

time	type	duration

NOTES

WEEK TWO

WEEKLY SUMMARY

BLOOD SUGAR

day	MORNING pre	MORNING post	SNACK pre	SNACK post	MIDDAY pre	MIDDAY post	SNACK pre	SNACK post	EVENING pre	EVENING post	NIGHT pre	NIGHT post
1												
2												
3												
4												
5												
6												
7												
AVG.												

MACROS

day	calories	fat	carbs	fiber	protein
1					
2					
3					
4					
5					
6					
7					
AVG.					

NOTES

ENERGY LEVEL AVERAGE

1 2 3 4 5 6 7 8 9 10

LOW ———— HIGH

STRESS LEVEL AVERAGE

1 2 3 4 5 6 7 8 9 10

LOW ———— HIGH

DAYS OF EXERCISE

1 2 3 4 5 6 7

AVG. MIN.

____

GOALS MET

ADJUSTMENTS

WEEK THREE

DAY ONE

date: ____________ S M T W T F S sleep hours: ________

fasting blood sugar: ____________ time: ________ am pm

MORNING

blood sugar: ________ time: ________ am pm

food/drink	calories	fat	carbs	fiber	protein
totals:					

medication: ____________ dose: ________ time: ________ am pm

post-meal blood sugar: ________ time: ________ am pm

SNACK

blood sugar: ________ time: ________ am pm

food/drink	calories	fat	carbs	fiber	protein

medication: ____________ dose: ________ time: ________ am pm

post-meal blood sugar: ________ time: ________ am pm

MIDDAY

blood sugar: ________ time: ________ am pm

food/drink	calories	fat	carbs	fiber	protein
totals:					

medication: ____________ dose: ________ time: ________ am pm

post-meal blood sugar: ________ time: ________ am pm

SNACK

blood sugar: ________ time: ________ am pm

food/drink	calories	fat	carbs	fiber	protein

medication: ____________ dose: ________ time: ________ am pm

post-meal blood sugar: ________ time: ________ am pm

EVENING blood sugar: ____________ time: ____________ am pm

food/drink	calories	fat	carbs	fiber	protein
totals:					

medication: ______________________ dose: ____________ time: ____________ am pm

post-meal blood sugar: ____________ time: ____________ am pm

NIGHT blood sugar: ____________ time: ____________ am pm

food/drink	calories	fat	carbs	fiber	protein

medication: ______________________ dose: ____________ time: ____________ am pm

post-meal blood sugar: ____________ time: ____________ am pm

AVG B.S. ____________

	calories	fat	carbs	fiber	protein
DAILY TOTALS					

ENERGY LEVEL

1 2 3 4 5 6 7 8 9 10

LOW ——————— HIGH

STRESS LEVEL

1 2 3 4 5 6 7 8 9 10

LOW ——————— HIGH

EXERCISE

time	type	duration

NOTES

DAY TWO

date: ________________ S M T W T F S sleep hours: ________

fasting blood sugar: ______________ time: ________ am pm

MORNING

blood sugar: __________ time: __________ am pm

food/drink	calories	fat	carbs	fiber	protein
totals:					

medication: ______________________ dose: ________ time: ________ am pm

post-meal blood sugar: __________ time: __________ am pm

SNACK

blood sugar: __________ time: __________ am pm

food/drink	calories	fat	carbs	fiber	protein

medication: ______________________ dose: ________ time: ________ am pm

post-meal blood sugar: __________ time: __________ am pm

MIDDAY

blood sugar: __________ time: __________ am pm

food/drink	calories	fat	carbs	fiber	protein
totals:					

medication: ______________________ dose: ________ time: ________ am pm

post-meal blood sugar: __________ time: __________ am pm

SNACK

blood sugar: __________ time: __________ am pm

food/drink	calories	fat	carbs	fiber	protein

medication: ______________________ dose: ________ time: ________ am pm

post-meal blood sugar: __________ time: __________ am pm

EVENING blood sugar: ______________ time: ______________ am pm

food/drink	calories	fat	carbs	fiber	protein
totals:					

medication: ______________________________ dose: ____________ time: __________ am pm

post-meal blood sugar: ______________ time: ______________ am pm

NIGHT blood sugar: ______________ time: ______________ am pm

food/drink	calories	fat	carbs	fiber	protein

medication: ______________________________ dose: ____________ time: __________ am pm

post-meal blood sugar: ______________ time: ______________ am pm

AVG B.S.	

	calories	fat	carbs	fiber	protein
DAILY TOTALS					

ENERGY LEVEL

1 2 3 4 5 6 7 8 9 10

LOW —— HIGH

STRESS LEVEL

1 2 3 4 5 6 7 8 9 10

LOW —— HIGH

EXERCISE

time	type	duration

NOTES

DAY THREE

date: ______________ S M T W T F S sleep hours: ________

fasting blood sugar: ______________ time: ________ am pm

MORNING blood sugar: ________ time: ________ am pm

food/drink	calories	fat	carbs	fiber	protein
totals:					

medication: ______________ dose: ________ time: ________ am pm

post-meal blood sugar: ________ time: ________ am pm

SNACK blood sugar: ________ time: ________ am pm

food/drink	calories	fat	carbs	fiber	protein

medication: ______________ dose: ________ time: ________ am pm

post-meal blood sugar: ________ time: ________ am pm

MIDDAY blood sugar: ________ time: ________ am pm

food/drink	calories	fat	carbs	fiber	protein
totals:					

medication: ______________ dose: ________ time: ________ am pm

post-meal blood sugar: ________ time: ________ am pm

SNACK blood sugar: ________ time: ________ am pm

food/drink	calories	fat	carbs	fiber	protein

medication: ______________ dose: ________ time: ________ am pm

post-meal blood sugar: ________ time: ________ am pm

EVENING blood sugar: ____________ time: ____________ am pm

food/drink	calories	fat	carbs	fiber	protein
totals:					

medication: ____________ dose: ____________ time: ____________ am pm

post-meal blood sugar: ____________ time: ____________ am pm

NIGHT blood sugar: ____________ time: ____________ am pm

food/drink	calories	fat	carbs	fiber	protein

medication: ____________ dose: ____________ time: ____________ am pm

post-meal blood sugar: ____________ time: ____________ am pm

AVG B.S. ____________

	calories	fat	carbs	fiber	protein
DAILY TOTALS					

ENERGY LEVEL

1 2 3 4 5 6 7 8 9 10

LOW —— HIGH

STRESS LEVEL

1 2 3 4 5 6 7 8 9 10

LOW —— HIGH

EXERCISE

time	type	duration

NOTES

DAY FOUR

date: ____________________ S M T W T F S sleep hours: __________

fasting blood sugar: ________________ time: ____________ am pm

MORNING blood sugar: ____________ time: ____________ am pm

food/drink	calories	fat	carbs	fiber	protein
totals:					

medication: ____________________________ dose: __________ time: _________ am pm

post-meal blood sugar: ____________ time: ____________ am pm

SNACK blood sugar: ____________ time: ____________ am pm

food/drink	calories	fat	carbs	fiber	protein

medication: ____________________________ dose: __________ time: _________ am pm

post-meal blood sugar: ____________ time: ____________ am pm

MIDDAY blood sugar: ____________ time: ____________ am pm

food/drink	calories	fat	carbs	fiber	protein
totals:					

medication: ____________________________ dose: __________ time: _________ am pm

post-meal blood sugar: ____________ time: ____________ am pm

SNACK blood sugar: ____________ time: ____________ am pm

food/drink	calories	fat	carbs	fiber	protein

medication: ____________________________ dose: __________ time: _________ am pm

post-meal blood sugar: ____________ time: ____________ am pm

EVENING blood sugar: ____________ time: ____________ am pm

food/drink	calories	fat	carbs	fiber	protein
totals:					

medication: ______________________ dose: __________ time: ________ am pm

post-meal blood sugar: ____________ time: ____________ am pm

NIGHT blood sugar: ____________ time: ____________ am pm

food/drink	calories	fat	carbs	fiber	protein

medication: ______________________ dose: __________ time: ________ am pm

post-meal blood sugar: ____________ time: ____________ am pm

AVG B.S.	

	calories	fat	carbs	fiber	protein
DAILY TOTALS					

ENERGY LEVEL

1 2 3 4 5 6 7 8 9 10

LOW ——— HIGH

STRESS LEVEL

1 2 3 4 5 6 7 8 9 10

LOW ——— HIGH

EXERCISE

time	type	duration

NOTES

DAY FIVE

date: ____________ S M T W T F S sleep hours: ________

fasting blood sugar: ____________ time: ________ am pm

MORNING

blood sugar: ________ time: ________ am pm

food/drink	calories	fat	carbs	fiber	protein
totals:					

medication: ____________ dose: ________ time: ________ am pm

post-meal blood sugar: ________ time: ________ am pm

SNACK

blood sugar: ________ time: ________ am pm

food/drink	calories	fat	carbs	fiber	protein

medication: ____________ dose: ________ time: ________ am pm

post-meal blood sugar: ________ time: ________ am pm

MIDDAY

blood sugar: ________ time: ________ am pm

food/drink	calories	fat	carbs	fiber	protein
totals:					

medication: ____________ dose: ________ time: ________ am pm

post-meal blood sugar: ________ time: ________ am pm

SNACK

blood sugar: ________ time: ________ am pm

food/drink	calories	fat	carbs	fiber	protein

medication: ____________ dose: ________ time: ________ am pm

post-meal blood sugar: ________ time: ________ am pm

EVENING blood sugar: ____________ time: ____________ am pm

food/drink	calories	fat	carbs	fiber	protein
totals:					

medication: ________________________ dose: __________ time: ________ am pm

post-meal blood sugar: ____________ time: ____________ am pm

NIGHT blood sugar: ____________ time: ____________ am pm

food/drink	calories	fat	carbs	fiber	protein

medication: ________________________ dose: __________ time: ________ am pm

post-meal blood sugar: ____________ time: ____________ am pm

AVG B.S.	

	calories	fat	carbs	fiber	protein
DAILY TOTALS					

ENERGY LEVEL

1 2 3 4 5 6 7 8 9 10

LOW ——— HIGH

STRESS LEVEL

1 2 3 4 5 6 7 8 9 10

LOW ——— HIGH

EXERCISE

time	type	duration

NOTES

DAY SIX

date: ____________ S M T W T F S sleep hours: ________

fasting blood sugar: ____________ time: ________ am pm

MORNING

blood sugar: ________ time: ________ am pm

food/drink	calories	fat	carbs	fiber	protein
totals:					

medication: ____________ dose: ________ time: ________ am pm

post-meal blood sugar: ________ time: ________ am pm

SNACK

blood sugar: ________ time: ________ am pm

food/drink	calories	fat	carbs	fiber	protein

medication: ____________ dose: ________ time: ________ am pm

post-meal blood sugar: ________ time: ________ am pm

MIDDAY

blood sugar: ________ time: ________ am pm

food/drink	calories	fat	carbs	fiber	protein
totals:					

medication: ____________ dose: ________ time: ________ am pm

post-meal blood sugar: ________ time: ________ am pm

SNACK

blood sugar: ________ time: ________ am pm

food/drink	calories	fat	carbs	fiber	protein

medication: ____________ dose: ________ time: ________ am pm

post-meal blood sugar: ________ time: ________ am pm

EVENING blood sugar: ______________ time: ______________ am pm

food/drink	calories	fat	carbs	fiber	protein
totals:					

medication: ______________________________ dose: ____________ time: __________ am pm

post-meal blood sugar: ______________ time: ______________ am pm

NIGHT blood sugar: ______________ time: ______________ am pm

food/drink	calories	fat	carbs	fiber	protein

medication: ______________________________ dose: ____________ time: __________ am pm

post-meal blood sugar: ______________ time: ______________ am pm

AVG B.S.	

	calories	fat	carbs	fiber	protein
DAILY TOTALS					

ENERGY LEVEL

1 2 3 4 5 6 7 8 9 10

LOW ———————— HIGH

STRESS LEVEL

1 2 3 4 5 6 7 8 9 10

LOW ———————— HIGH

EXERCISE

time	type	duration

NOTES

DAY SEVEN

date: ____________ S M T W T F S sleep hours: ________

fasting blood sugar: ____________ time: ________ am pm

MORNING blood sugar: ________ time: ________ am pm

food/drink	calories	fat	carbs	fiber	protein
totals:					

medication: ____________ dose: ________ time: ________ am pm

post-meal blood sugar: ________ time: ________ am pm

SNACK blood sugar: ________ time: ________ am pm

food/drink	calories	fat	carbs	fiber	protein

medication: ____________ dose: ________ time: ________ am pm

post-meal blood sugar: ________ time: ________ am pm

MIDDAY blood sugar: ________ time: ________ am pm

food/drink	calories	fat	carbs	fiber	protein
totals:					

medication: ____________ dose: ________ time: ________ am pm

post-meal blood sugar: ________ time: ________ am pm

SNACK blood sugar: ________ time: ________ am pm

food/drink	calories	fat	carbs	fiber	protein

medication: ____________ dose: ________ time: ________ am pm

post-meal blood sugar: ________ time: ________ am pm

EVENING blood sugar: ____________ time: ____________ am pm

food/drink	calories	fat	carbs	fiber	protein
totals:					

medication: __________________________ dose: __________ time: ________ am pm

post-meal blood sugar: ____________ time: ____________ am pm

NIGHT blood sugar: ____________ time: ____________ am pm

food/drink	calories	fat	carbs	fiber	protein

medication: __________________________ dose: __________ time: ________ am pm

post-meal blood sugar: ____________ time: ____________ am pm

AVG B.S.	

	calories	fat	carbs	fiber	protein
DAILY TOTALS					

ENERGY LEVEL

1 2 3 4 5 6 7 8 9 10

LOW ———————— HIGH

STRESS LEVEL

1 2 3 4 5 6 7 8 9 10

LOW ———————— HIGH

EXERCISE

time	type	duration

NOTES

WEEK THREE

WEEKLY SUMMARY

BLOOD SUGAR

	MORNING		SNACK		MIDDAY		SNACK		EVENING		NIGHT	
day	pre	post	pre	post	pre	post	pre	post	pre	post	pre	post
1												
2												
3												
4												
5												
6												
7												
AVG.												

MACROS

day	calories	fat	carbs	fiber	protein
1					
2					
3					
4					
5					
6					
7					
AVG.					

NOTES

ENERGY LEVEL AVERAGE

1 2 3 4 5 6 7 8 9 10

LOW —— HIGH

STRESS LEVEL AVERAGE

1 2 3 4 5 6 7 8 9 10

LOW —— HIGH

DAYS OF EXERCISE

1 2 3 4 5 6 7

AVG. MIN.

____

GOALS MET

ADJUSTMENTS

WEEK FOUR

DAY ONE

date: ______________ S M T W T F S sleep hours: __________

fasting blood sugar: ______________ time: __________ am pm

MORNING blood sugar: __________ time: __________ am pm

food/drink	calories	fat	carbs	fiber	protein
totals:					

medication: ______________ dose: __________ time: __________ am pm

post-meal blood sugar: __________ time: __________ am pm

SNACK blood sugar: __________ time: __________ am pm

food/drink	calories	fat	carbs	fiber	protein

medication: ______________ dose: __________ time: __________ am pm

post-meal blood sugar: __________ time: __________ am pm

MIDDAY blood sugar: __________ time: __________ am pm

food/drink	calories	fat	carbs	fiber	protein
totals:					

medication: ______________ dose: __________ time: __________ am pm

post-meal blood sugar: __________ time: __________ am pm

SNACK blood sugar: __________ time: __________ am pm

food/drink	calories	fat	carbs	fiber	protein

medication: ______________ dose: __________ time: __________ am pm

post-meal blood sugar: __________ time: __________ am pm

EVENING blood sugar: ________ time: ________ am pm

food/drink	calories	fat	carbs	fiber	protein
totals:					

medication: ________ dose: ________ time: ________ am pm

post-meal blood sugar: ________ time: ________ am pm

NIGHT blood sugar: ________ time: ________ am pm

food/drink	calories	fat	carbs	fiber	protein

medication: ________ dose: ________ time: ________ am pm

post-meal blood sugar: ________ time: ________ am pm

AVG B.S.	

	calories	fat	carbs	fiber	protein
DAILY TOTALS					

ENERGY LEVEL

1 2 3 4 5 6 7 8 9 10

LOW —— HIGH

STRESS LEVEL

1 2 3 4 5 6 7 8 9 10

LOW —— HIGH

EXERCISE

time	type	duration

NOTES

DAY TWO

date: ____________________ S M T W T F S sleep hours: __________

fasting blood sugar: ________________ time: ____________ am pm

MORNING blood sugar: ____________ time: ____________ am pm

food/drink	calories	fat	carbs	fiber	protein
totals:					

medication: ____________________________ dose: __________ time: _________ am pm

post-meal blood sugar: ____________ time: ____________ am pm

SNACK blood sugar: ____________ time: ____________ am pm

food/drink	calories	fat	carbs	fiber	protein

medication: ____________________________ dose: __________ time: _________ am pm

post-meal blood sugar: ____________ time: ____________ am pm

MIDDAY blood sugar: ____________ time: ____________ am pm

food/drink	calories	fat	carbs	fiber	protein
totals:					

medication: ____________________________ dose: __________ time: _________ am pm

post-meal blood sugar: ____________ time: ____________ am pm

SNACK blood sugar: ____________ time: ____________ am pm

food/drink	calories	fat	carbs	fiber	protein

medication: ____________________________ dose: __________ time: _________ am pm

post-meal blood sugar: ____________ time: ____________ am pm

EVENING	blood sugar: ______	time: ______ am/pm			
food/drink	calories	fat	carbs	fiber	protein
totals:					

medication: ______________ dose: ______ time: ______ am pm

post-meal blood sugar: ______ time: ______ am pm

NIGHT	blood sugar: ______	time: ______ am/pm			
food/drink	calories	fat	carbs	fiber	protein

medication: ______________ dose: ______ time: ______ am pm

post-meal blood sugar: ______ time: ______ am pm

AVG B.S.	

	calories	fat	carbs	fiber	protein
DAILY TOTALS					

ENERGY LEVEL

1 2 3 4 5 6 7 8 9 10

LOW ——— HIGH

STRESS LEVEL

1 2 3 4 5 6 7 8 9 10

LOW ——— HIGH

EXERCISE

time	type	duration

NOTES

DAY THREE

date: ____________ S M T W T F S sleep hours: ________

fasting blood sugar: ____________ time: ________ am pm

MORNING blood sugar: ________ time: ________ am pm

food/drink	calories	fat	carbs	fiber	protein
totals:					

medication: ____________ dose: ________ time: ________ am pm

post-meal blood sugar: ________ time: ________ am pm

SNACK blood sugar: ________ time: ________ am pm

food/drink	calories	fat	carbs	fiber	protein

medication: ____________ dose: ________ time: ________ am pm

post-meal blood sugar: ________ time: ________ am pm

MIDDAY blood sugar: ________ time: ________ am pm

food/drink	calories	fat	carbs	fiber	protein
totals:					

medication: ____________ dose: ________ time: ________ am pm

post-meal blood sugar: ________ time: ________ am pm

SNACK blood sugar: ________ time: ________ am pm

food/drink	calories	fat	carbs	fiber	protein

medication: ____________ dose: ________ time: ________ am pm

post-meal blood sugar: ________ time: ________ am pm

EVENING blood sugar: ____________ time: ____________ am pm

food/drink	calories	fat	carbs	fiber	protein
totals:					

medication: ______________________ dose: __________ time: ________ am pm

post-meal blood sugar: ____________ time: ____________ am pm

NIGHT blood sugar: ____________ time: ____________ am pm

food/drink	calories	fat	carbs	fiber	protein

medication: ______________________ dose: __________ time: ________ am pm

post-meal blood sugar: ____________ time: ____________ am pm

AVG B.S.	

	calories	fat	carbs	fiber	protein
DAILY TOTALS					

ENERGY LEVEL

1 2 3 4 5 6 7 8 9 10

LOW ———————— HIGH

STRESS LEVEL

1 2 3 4 5 6 7 8 9 10

LOW ———————— HIGH

EXERCISE

time	type	duration

NOTES

DAY FOUR

date: ____________ S M T W T F S sleep hours: ________

fasting blood sugar: ____________ time: ________ am pm

MORNING blood sugar: ________ time: ________ am pm

food/drink	calories	fat	carbs	fiber	protein
totals:					

medication: ____________ dose: ________ time: ________ am pm

post-meal blood sugar: ________ time: ________ am pm

SNACK blood sugar: ________ time: ________ am pm

food/drink	calories	fat	carbs	fiber	protein

medication: ____________ dose: ________ time: ________ am pm

post-meal blood sugar: ________ time: ________ am pm

MIDDAY blood sugar: ________ time: ________ am pm

food/drink	calories	fat	carbs	fiber	protein
totals:					

medication: ____________ dose: ________ time: ________ am pm

post-meal blood sugar: ________ time: ________ am pm

SNACK blood sugar: ________ time: ________ am pm

food/drink	calories	fat	carbs	fiber	protein

medication: ____________ dose: ________ time: ________ am pm

post-meal blood sugar: ________ time: ________ am pm

EVENING blood sugar: ______________ time: ______________ am pm

food/drink	calories	fat	carbs	fiber	protein
totals:					

medication: ______________ dose: ______________ time: ______________ am pm

post-meal blood sugar: ______________ time: ______________ am pm

NIGHT blood sugar: ______________ time: ______________ am pm

food/drink	calories	fat	carbs	fiber	protein

medication: ______________ dose: ______________ time: ______________ am pm

post-meal blood sugar: ______________ time: ______________ am pm

AVG B.S.	

	calories	fat	carbs	fiber	protein
DAILY TOTALS					

ENERGY LEVEL

1 2 3 4 5 6 7 8 9 10

LOW —————————— HIGH

STRESS LEVEL

1 2 3 4 5 6 7 8 9 10

LOW —————————— HIGH

EXERCISE

time	type	duration

NOTES

DAY FIVE

date: ____________ S M T W T F S sleep hours: ________

fasting blood sugar: ____________ time: ________ am pm

MORNING blood sugar: ________ time: ________ am pm

food/drink	calories	fat	carbs	fiber	protein
totals:					

medication: ________________ dose: ________ time: ________ am pm

post-meal blood sugar: ________ time: ________ am pm

SNACK blood sugar: ________ time: ________ am pm

food/drink	calories	fat	carbs	fiber	protein

medication: ________________ dose: ________ time: ________ am pm

post-meal blood sugar: ________ time: ________ am pm

MIDDAY blood sugar: ________ time: ________ am pm

food/drink	calories	fat	carbs	fiber	protein
totals:					

medication: ________________ dose: ________ time: ________ am pm

post-meal blood sugar: ________ time: ________ am pm

SNACK blood sugar: ________ time: ________ am pm

food/drink	calories	fat	carbs	fiber	protein

medication: ________________ dose: ________ time: ________ am pm

post-meal blood sugar: ________ time: ________ am pm

EVENING blood sugar: ____________ time: ____________ am pm

food/drink	calories	fat	carbs	fiber	protein
totals:					

medication: ______________________ dose: __________ time: __________ am pm

post-meal blood sugar: ____________ time: ____________ am pm

NIGHT blood sugar: ____________ time: ____________ am pm

food/drink	calories	fat	carbs	fiber	protein

medication: ______________________ dose: __________ time: __________ am pm

post-meal blood sugar: ____________ time: ____________ am pm

AVG B.S.	

	calories	fat	carbs	fiber	protein
DAILY TOTALS					

ENERGY LEVEL

1 2 3 4 5 6 7 8 9 10

LOW ——— HIGH

STRESS LEVEL

1 2 3 4 5 6 7 8 9 10

LOW ——— HIGH

EXERCISE

time	type	duration

NOTES

DAY SIX

date: ____________ S M T W T F S sleep hours: ________

fasting blood sugar: ____________ time: ________ am pm

MORNING blood sugar: ________ time: ________ am pm

food/drink	calories	fat	carbs	fiber	protein
totals:					

medication: ____________ dose: ________ time: ________ am pm

post-meal blood sugar: ________ time: ________ am pm

SNACK blood sugar: ________ time: ________ am pm

food/drink	calories	fat	carbs	fiber	protein

medication: ____________ dose: ________ time: ________ am pm

post-meal blood sugar: ________ time: ________ am pm

MIDDAY blood sugar: ________ time: ________ am pm

food/drink	calories	fat	carbs	fiber	protein
totals:					

medication: ____________ dose: ________ time: ________ am pm

post-meal blood sugar: ________ time: ________ am pm

SNACK blood sugar: ________ time: ________ am pm

food/drink	calories	fat	carbs	fiber	protein

medication: ____________ dose: ________ time: ________ am pm

post-meal blood sugar: ________ time: ________ am pm

EVENING	blood sugar: ______	time: ______ am pm			
food/drink	calories	fat	carbs	fiber	protein
totals:					

medication: ______ dose: ______ time: ______ am pm

post-meal blood sugar: ______ time: ______ am pm

NIGHT	blood sugar: ______	time: ______ am pm			
food/drink	calories	fat	carbs	fiber	protein

medication: ______ dose: ______ time: ______ am pm

post-meal blood sugar: ______ time: ______ am pm

AVG B.S.	

	calories	fat	carbs	fiber	protein
DAILY TOTALS					

ENERGY LEVEL

1 2 3 4 5 6 7 8 9 10

LOW —— HIGH

STRESS LEVEL

1 2 3 4 5 6 7 8 9 10

LOW —— HIGH

EXERCISE

time	type	duration

NOTES

DAY SEVEN

date: ____________ S M T W T F S sleep hours: ______

fasting blood sugar: ____________ time: ________ am pm

MORNING blood sugar: ________ time: ________ am pm

food/drink	calories	fat	carbs	fiber	protein
totals:					

medication: ____________ dose: ______ time: ______ am pm

post-meal blood sugar: ________ time: ________ am pm

SNACK blood sugar: ________ time: ________ am pm

food/drink	calories	fat	carbs	fiber	protein

medication: ____________ dose: ______ time: ______ am pm

post-meal blood sugar: ________ time: ________ am pm

MIDDAY blood sugar: ________ time: ________ am pm

food/drink	calories	fat	carbs	fiber	protein
totals:					

medication: ____________ dose: ______ time: ______ am pm

post-meal blood sugar: ________ time: ________ am pm

SNACK blood sugar: ________ time: ________ am pm

food/drink	calories	fat	carbs	fiber	protein

medication: ____________ dose: ______ time: ______ am pm

post-meal blood sugar: ________ time: ________ am pm

EVENING blood sugar: ________ time: ________ am/pm

food/drink	calories	fat	carbs	fiber	protein
totals:					

medication: ____________ dose: ________ time: ________ am/pm

post-meal blood sugar: ________ time: ________ am/pm

NIGHT blood sugar: ________ time: ________ am/pm

food/drink	calories	fat	carbs	fiber	protein

medication: ____________ dose: ________ time: ________ am/pm

post-meal blood sugar: ________ time: ________ am/pm

AVG B.S.	

	calories	fat	carbs	fiber	protein
DAILY TOTALS					

ENERGY LEVEL

1 2 3 4 5 6 7 8 9 10

LOW ——— HIGH

STRESS LEVEL

1 2 3 4 5 6 7 8 9 10

LOW ——— HIGH

EXERCISE

time	type	duration

NOTES

WEEK FOUR

WEEKLY SUMMARY

BLOOD SUGAR

day	MORNING pre	MORNING post	SNACK pre	SNACK post	MIDDAY pre	MIDDAY post	SNACK pre	SNACK post	EVENING pre	EVENING post	NIGHT pre	NIGHT post
1												
2												
3												
4												
5												
6												
7												
AVG.												

MACROS

day	calories	fat	carbs	fiber	protein
1					
2					
3					
4					
5					
6					
7					
AVG.					

NOTES

ENERGY LEVEL AVERAGE

1 2 3 4 5 6 7 8 9 10

LOW —— HIGH

STRESS LEVEL AVERAGE

1 2 3 4 5 6 7 8 9 10

LOW —— HIGH

DAYS OF EXERCISE

1 2 3 4 5 6 7

AVG. MIN.

______

GOALS MET

ADJUSTMENTS

WEEK FIVE

DAY ONE

date: ____________ S M T W T F S sleep hours: ________

fasting blood sugar: ____________ time: ________ am pm

MORNING

blood sugar: ________ time: ________ am pm

food/drink	calories	fat	carbs	fiber	protein
totals:					

medication: ____________ dose: ________ time: ________ am pm

post-meal blood sugar: ________ time: ________ am pm

SNACK

blood sugar: ________ time: ________ am pm

food/drink	calories	fat	carbs	fiber	protein

medication: ____________ dose: ________ time: ________ am pm

post-meal blood sugar: ________ time: ________ am pm

MIDDAY

blood sugar: ________ time: ________ am pm

food/drink	calories	fat	carbs	fiber	protein
totals:					

medication: ____________ dose: ________ time: ________ am pm

post-meal blood sugar: ________ time: ________ am pm

SNACK

blood sugar: ________ time: ________ am pm

food/drink	calories	fat	carbs	fiber	protein

medication: ____________ dose: ________ time: ________ am pm

post-meal blood sugar: ________ time: ________ am pm

EVENING

blood sugar: ____________ time: ____________ am pm

food/drink	calories	fat	carbs	fiber	protein
totals:					

medication: ____________________ dose: ____________ time: ____________ am pm

post-meal blood sugar: ____________ time: ____________ am pm

NIGHT

blood sugar: ____________ time: ____________ am pm

food/drink	calories	fat	carbs	fiber	protein

medication: ____________________ dose: ____________ time: ____________ am pm

post-meal blood sugar: ____________ time: ____________ am pm

AVG B.S.	

	calories	fat	carbs	fiber	protein
DAILY TOTALS					

ENERGY LEVEL

1 2 3 4 5 6 7 8 9 10

LOW —————— HIGH

STRESS LEVEL

1 2 3 4 5 6 7 8 9 10

LOW —————— HIGH

EXERCISE

time	type	duration

NOTES

DAY TWO

date: ____________ S M T W T F S sleep hours: ________

fasting blood sugar: ____________ time: ________ am pm

MORNING

blood sugar: ________ time: ________ am pm

food/drink	calories	fat	carbs	fiber	protein
totals:					

medication: ____________ dose: ________ time: ________ am pm

post-meal blood sugar: ________ time: ________ am pm

SNACK

blood sugar: ________ time: ________ am pm

food/drink	calories	fat	carbs	fiber	protein

medication: ____________ dose: ________ time: ________ am pm

post-meal blood sugar: ________ time: ________ am pm

MIDDAY

blood sugar: ________ time: ________ am pm

food/drink	calories	fat	carbs	fiber	protein
totals:					

medication: ____________ dose: ________ time: ________ am pm

post-meal blood sugar: ________ time: ________ am pm

SNACK

blood sugar: ________ time: ________ am pm

food/drink	calories	fat	carbs	fiber	protein

medication: ____________ dose: ________ time: ________ am pm

post-meal blood sugar: ________ time: ________ am pm

EVENING	blood sugar: ______	time: ______ am/pm			
food/drink	calories	fat	carbs	fiber	protein
totals:					

medication: ______ dose: ______ time: ______ am pm

post-meal blood sugar: ______ time: ______ am pm

NIGHT	blood sugar: ______	time: ______ am/pm			
food/drink	calories	fat	carbs	fiber	protein

medication: ______ dose: ______ time: ______ am pm

post-meal blood sugar: ______ time: ______ am pm

AVG B.S.	

	calories	fat	carbs	fiber	protein
DAILY TOTALS					

ENERGY LEVEL

1 2 3 4 5 6 7 8 9 10

LOW —— HIGH

STRESS LEVEL

1 2 3 4 5 6 7 8 9 10

LOW —— HIGH

EXERCISE

time	type	duration

NOTES

DAY THREE

date: ____________ S M T W T F S sleep hours: ________

fasting blood sugar: ____________ time: ________ am pm

MORNING blood sugar: ________ time: ________ am pm

food/drink	calories	fat	carbs	fiber	protein
totals:					

medication: ____________ dose: ________ time: ________ am pm

post-meal blood sugar: ________ time: ________ am pm

SNACK blood sugar: ________ time: ________ am pm

food/drink	calories	fat	carbs	fiber	protein

medication: ____________ dose: ________ time: ________ am pm

post-meal blood sugar: ________ time: ________ am pm

MIDDAY blood sugar: ________ time: ________ am pm

food/drink	calories	fat	carbs	fiber	protein
totals:					

medication: ____________ dose: ________ time: ________ am pm

post-meal blood sugar: ________ time: ________ am pm

SNACK blood sugar: ________ time: ________ am pm

food/drink	calories	fat	carbs	fiber	protein

medication: ____________ dose: ________ time: ________ am pm

post-meal blood sugar: ________ time: ________ am pm

EVENING

blood sugar: ____________ time: ____________ am pm

food/drink	calories	fat	carbs	fiber	protein
totals:					

medication: ____________ dose: ____________ time: ____________ am pm

post-meal blood sugar: ____________ time: ____________ am pm

NIGHT

blood sugar: ____________ time: ____________ am pm

food/drink	calories	fat	carbs	fiber	protein

medication: ____________ dose: ____________ time: ____________ am pm

post-meal blood sugar: ____________ time: ____________ am pm

AVG B.S.	

	calories	fat	carbs	fiber	protein
DAILY TOTALS					

ENERGY LEVEL

1 2 3 4 5 6 7 8 9 10

LOW ——— HIGH

STRESS LEVEL

1 2 3 4 5 6 7 8 9 10

LOW ——— HIGH

EXERCISE

time	type	duration

NOTES

DAY FOUR

date: ____________ S M T W T F S sleep hours: ________

fasting blood sugar: ____________ time: ________ am pm

MORNING

blood sugar: ________ time: ________ am pm

food/drink	calories	fat	carbs	fiber	protein
totals:					

medication: ____________ dose: ________ time: ________ am pm

post-meal blood sugar: ________ time: ________ am pm

SNACK

blood sugar: ________ time: ________ am pm

food/drink	calories	fat	carbs	fiber	protein

medication: ____________ dose: ________ time: ________ am pm

post-meal blood sugar: ________ time: ________ am pm

MIDDAY

blood sugar: ________ time: ________ am pm

food/drink	calories	fat	carbs	fiber	protein
totals:					

medication: ____________ dose: ________ time: ________ am pm

post-meal blood sugar: ________ time: ________ am pm

SNACK

blood sugar: ________ time: ________ am pm

food/drink	calories	fat	carbs	fiber	protein

medication: ____________ dose: ________ time: ________ am pm

post-meal blood sugar: ________ time: ________ am pm

EVENING blood sugar: ____________ time: ____________ am/pm

food/drink	calories	fat	carbs	fiber	protein
totals:					

medication: ______________________ dose: __________ time: __________ am/pm

post-meal blood sugar: ____________ time: ____________ am/pm

NIGHT blood sugar: ____________ time: ____________ am/pm

food/drink	calories	fat	carbs	fiber	protein

medication: ______________________ dose: __________ time: __________ am/pm

post-meal blood sugar: ____________ time: ____________ am/pm

AVG B.S. ________

	calories	fat	carbs	fiber	protein
DAILY TOTALS					

ENERGY LEVEL

1 2 3 4 5 6 7 8 9 10

LOW ———————— HIGH

STRESS LEVEL

1 2 3 4 5 6 7 8 9 10

LOW ———————— HIGH

EXERCISE

time	type	duration

NOTES

DAY FIVE

date: ______________ S M T W T F S sleep hours: ________

fasting blood sugar: ______________ time: ________ am pm

MORNING

blood sugar: ________ time: ________ am pm

food/drink	calories	fat	carbs	fiber	protein
totals:					

medication: ______________ dose: ________ time: ________ am pm

post-meal blood sugar: ________ time: ________ am pm

SNACK

blood sugar: ________ time: ________ am pm

food/drink	calories	fat	carbs	fiber	protein

medication: ______________ dose: ________ time: ________ am pm

post-meal blood sugar: ________ time: ________ am pm

MIDDAY

blood sugar: ________ time: ________ am pm

food/drink	calories	fat	carbs	fiber	protein
totals:					

medication: ______________ dose: ________ time: ________ am pm

post-meal blood sugar: ________ time: ________ am pm

SNACK

blood sugar: ________ time: ________ am pm

food/drink	calories	fat	carbs	fiber	protein

medication: ______________ dose: ________ time: ________ am pm

post-meal blood sugar: ________ time: ________ am pm

EVENING	blood sugar: ______	time: ______ am/pm			
food/drink	calories	fat	carbs	fiber	protein
totals:					

medication: ______ dose: ______ time: ______ am pm

post-meal blood sugar: ______ time: ______ am pm

NIGHT	blood sugar: ______	time: ______ am/pm			
food/drink	calories	fat	carbs	fiber	protein

medication: ______ dose: ______ time: ______ am pm

post-meal blood sugar: ______ time: ______ am pm

AVG B.S.	

	calories	fat	carbs	fiber	protein
DAILY TOTALS					

ENERGY LEVEL

1 2 3 4 5 6 7 8 9 10

LOW ———— HIGH

STRESS LEVEL

1 2 3 4 5 6 7 8 9 10

LOW ———— HIGH

EXERCISE

time	type	duration

NOTES

DAY SIX

date: ____________ S M T W T F S sleep hours: ________

fasting blood sugar: ____________ time: ________ am pm

MORNING

blood sugar: ________ time: ________ am pm

food/drink	calories	fat	carbs	fiber	protein
totals:					

medication: ________________ dose: ________ time: ________ am pm

post-meal blood sugar: ________ time: ________ am pm

SNACK

blood sugar: ________ time: ________ am pm

food/drink	calories	fat	carbs	fiber	protein

medication: ________________ dose: ________ time: ________ am pm

post-meal blood sugar: ________ time: ________ am pm

MIDDAY

blood sugar: ________ time: ________ am pm

food/drink	calories	fat	carbs	fiber	protein
totals:					

medication: ________________ dose: ________ time: ________ am pm

post-meal blood sugar: ________ time: ________ am pm

SNACK

blood sugar: ________ time: ________ am pm

food/drink	calories	fat	carbs	fiber	protein

medication: ________________ dose: ________ time: ________ am pm

post-meal blood sugar: ________ time: ________ am pm

EVENING blood sugar: ____________ time: ____________ am pm

food/drink	calories	fat	carbs	fiber	protein
totals:					

medication: ____________________ dose: __________ time: __________ am pm

post-meal blood sugar: ____________ time: ____________ am pm

NIGHT blood sugar: ____________ time: ____________ am pm

food/drink	calories	fat	carbs	fiber	protein

medication: ____________________ dose: __________ time: __________ am pm

post-meal blood sugar: ____________ time: ____________ am pm

AVG B.S.	

	calories	fat	carbs	fiber	protein
DAILY TOTALS					

ENERGY LEVEL

1 2 3 4 5 6 7 8 9 10

LOW ——— HIGH

STRESS LEVEL

1 2 3 4 5 6 7 8 9 10

LOW ——— HIGH

EXERCISE

time	type	duration

NOTES

DAY SEVEN

date: ______________ S M T W T F S sleep hours: __________

fasting blood sugar: ______________ time: __________ am pm

MORNING blood sugar: __________ time: __________ am pm

food/drink	calories	fat	carbs	fiber	protein
totals:					

medication: ______________ dose: __________ time: __________ am pm

post-meal blood sugar: __________ time: __________ am pm

SNACK blood sugar: __________ time: __________ am pm

food/drink	calories	fat	carbs	fiber	protein

medication: ______________ dose: __________ time: __________ am pm

post-meal blood sugar: __________ time: __________ am pm

MIDDAY blood sugar: __________ time: __________ am pm

food/drink	calories	fat	carbs	fiber	protein
totals:					

medication: ______________ dose: __________ time: __________ am pm

post-meal blood sugar: __________ time: __________ am pm

SNACK blood sugar: __________ time: __________ am pm

food/drink	calories	fat	carbs	fiber	protein

medication: ______________ dose: __________ time: __________ am pm

post-meal blood sugar: __________ time: __________ am pm

EVENING	blood sugar: ______	time: ______ am pm			
food/drink	calories	fat	carbs	fiber	protein
totals:					

medication: ______ dose: ______ time: ______ am pm

post-meal blood sugar: ______ time: ______ am pm

NIGHT	blood sugar: ______	time: ______ am pm			
food/drink	calories	fat	carbs	fiber	protein

medication: ______ dose: ______ time: ______ am pm

post-meal blood sugar: ______ time: ______ am pm

AVG B.S.	

	calories	fat	carbs	fiber	protein
DAILY TOTALS					

ENERGY LEVEL

1 2 3 4 5 6 7 8 9 10

LOW — HIGH

STRESS LEVEL

1 2 3 4 5 6 7 8 9 10

LOW — HIGH

EXERCISE

time	type	duration

NOTES

WEEK FIVE

WEEKLY SUMMARY

BLOOD SUGAR

day	MORNING pre	MORNING post	SNACK pre	SNACK post	MIDDAY pre	MIDDAY post	SNACK pre	SNACK post	EVENING pre	EVENING post	NIGHT pre	NIGHT post
1												
2												
3												
4												
5												
6												
7												
AVG.												

MACROS

day	calories	fat	carbs	fiber	protein
1					
2					
3					
4					
5					
6					
7					
AVG.					

NOTES

ENERGY LEVEL AVERAGE

1 2 3 4 5 6 7 8 9 10

LOW —— HIGH

STRESS LEVEL AVERAGE

1 2 3 4 5 6 7 8 9 10

LOW —— HIGH

DAYS OF EXERCISE

1 2 3 4 5 6 7

AVG. MIN.

______

GOALS MET

ADJUSTMENTS

WEEK SIX

DAY ONE

date: ____________ S M T W T F S sleep hours: ________

fasting blood sugar: ____________ time: ________ am pm

MORNING blood sugar: ________ time: ________ am pm

food/drink	calories	fat	carbs	fiber	protein
totals:					

medication: ____________ dose: ________ time: ________ am pm

post-meal blood sugar: ________ time: ________ am pm

SNACK blood sugar: ________ time: ________ am pm

food/drink	calories	fat	carbs	fiber	protein

medication: ____________ dose: ________ time: ________ am pm

post-meal blood sugar: ________ time: ________ am pm

MIDDAY blood sugar: ________ time: ________ am pm

food/drink	calories	fat	carbs	fiber	protein
totals:					

medication: ____________ dose: ________ time: ________ am pm

post-meal blood sugar: ________ time: ________ am pm

SNACK blood sugar: ________ time: ________ am pm

food/drink	calories	fat	carbs	fiber	protein

medication: ____________ dose: ________ time: ________ am pm

post-meal blood sugar: ________ time: ________ am pm

EVENING blood sugar: ____________ time: ____________ am pm

food/drink	calories	fat	carbs	fiber	protein
totals:					

medication: ______________________ dose: ____________ time: ____________ am pm

post-meal blood sugar: ____________ time: ____________ am pm

NIGHT blood sugar: ____________ time: ____________ am pm

food/drink	calories	fat	carbs	fiber	protein

medication: ______________________ dose: ____________ time: ____________ am pm

post-meal blood sugar: ____________ time: ____________ am pm

AVG B.S.	

	calories	fat	carbs	fiber	protein
DAILY TOTALS					

ENERGY LEVEL

1 2 3 4 5 6 7 8 9 10

LOW ——— HIGH

STRESS LEVEL

1 2 3 4 5 6 7 8 9 10

LOW ——— HIGH

EXERCISE

time	type	duration

NOTES

DAY TWO

date: ____________ S M T W T F S sleep hours: ________

fasting blood sugar: ____________ time: ________ am pm

MORNING blood sugar: ________ time: ________ am pm

food/drink	calories	fat	carbs	fiber	protein
totals:					

medication: ____________ dose: ________ time: ________ am pm

post-meal blood sugar: ________ time: ________ am pm

SNACK blood sugar: ________ time: ________ am pm

food/drink	calories	fat	carbs	fiber	protein

medication: ____________ dose: ________ time: ________ am pm

post-meal blood sugar: ________ time: ________ am pm

MIDDAY blood sugar: ________ time: ________ am pm

food/drink	calories	fat	carbs	fiber	protein
totals:					

medication: ____________ dose: ________ time: ________ am pm

post-meal blood sugar: ________ time: ________ am pm

SNACK blood sugar: ________ time: ________ am pm

food/drink	calories	fat	carbs	fiber	protein

medication: ____________ dose: ________ time: ________ am pm

post-meal blood sugar: ________ time: ________ am pm

EVENING	blood sugar: ______	time: ______ am pm			
food/drink	calories	fat	carbs	fiber	protein
totals:					

medication: ______ dose: ______ time: ______ am pm

post-meal blood sugar: ______ time: ______ am pm

NIGHT	blood sugar: ______	time: ______ am pm			
food/drink	calories	fat	carbs	fiber	protein

medication: ______ dose: ______ time: ______ am pm

post-meal blood sugar: ______ time: ______ am pm

AVG B.S.	

	calories	fat	carbs	fiber	protein
DAILY TOTALS					

ENERGY LEVEL

1 2 3 4 5 6 7 8 9 10

LOW —— HIGH

STRESS LEVEL

1 2 3 4 5 6 7 8 9 10

LOW —— HIGH

EXERCISE

time	type	duration

NOTES

DAY THREE

date: ____________ S M T W T F S sleep hours: ________

fasting blood sugar: ____________ time: ________ am pm

MORNING

blood sugar: ________ time: ________ am pm

food/drink	calories	fat	carbs	fiber	protein
totals:					

medication: ____________ dose: ________ time: ________ am pm

post-meal blood sugar: ________ time: ________ am pm

SNACK

blood sugar: ________ time: ________ am pm

food/drink	calories	fat	carbs	fiber	protein

medication: ____________ dose: ________ time: ________ am pm

post-meal blood sugar: ________ time: ________ am pm

MIDDAY

blood sugar: ________ time: ________ am pm

food/drink	calories	fat	carbs	fiber	protein
totals:					

medication: ____________ dose: ________ time: ________ am pm

post-meal blood sugar: ________ time: ________ am pm

SNACK

blood sugar: ________ time: ________ am pm

food/drink	calories	fat	carbs	fiber	protein

medication: ____________ dose: ________ time: ________ am pm

post-meal blood sugar: ________ time: ________ am pm

EVENING blood sugar: ________ time: ________ am pm

food/drink	calories	fat	carbs	fiber	protein
totals:					

medication: ________ dose: ________ time: ________ am pm

post-meal blood sugar: ________ time: ________ am pm

NIGHT blood sugar: ________ time: ________ am pm

food/drink	calories	fat	carbs	fiber	protein

medication: ________ dose: ________ time: ________ am pm

post-meal blood sugar: ________ time: ________ am pm

AVG B.S.	

	calories	fat	carbs	fiber	protein
DAILY TOTALS					

ENERGY LEVEL

1 2 3 4 5 6 7 8 9 10

LOW —— HIGH

STRESS LEVEL

1 2 3 4 5 6 7 8 9 10

LOW —— HIGH

EXERCISE

time	type	duration

NOTES

DAY FOUR

date: ____________ S M T W T F S sleep hours: ________

fasting blood sugar: ____________ time: ________ am pm

MORNING

blood sugar: ________ time: ________ am pm

food/drink	calories	fat	carbs	fiber	protein
totals:					

medication: ____________ dose: ________ time: ________ am pm

post-meal blood sugar: ________ time: ________ am pm

SNACK

blood sugar: ________ time: ________ am pm

food/drink	calories	fat	carbs	fiber	protein

medication: ____________ dose: ________ time: ________ am pm

post-meal blood sugar: ________ time: ________ am pm

MIDDAY

blood sugar: ________ time: ________ am pm

food/drink	calories	fat	carbs	fiber	protein
totals:					

medication: ____________ dose: ________ time: ________ am pm

post-meal blood sugar: ________ time: ________ am pm

SNACK

blood sugar: ________ time: ________ am pm

food/drink	calories	fat	carbs	fiber	protein

medication: ____________ dose: ________ time: ________ am pm

post-meal blood sugar: ________ time: ________ am pm

EVENING	blood sugar: ______	time: ______ am pm

food/drink	calories	fat	carbs	fiber	protein
totals:					

medication: ______ dose: ______ time: ______ am pm

post-meal blood sugar: ______ time: ______ am pm

NIGHT	blood sugar: ______	time: ______ am pm

food/drink	calories	fat	carbs	fiber	protein

medication: ______ dose: ______ time: ______ am pm

post-meal blood sugar: ______ time: ______ am pm

AVG B.S.	

	calories	fat	carbs	fiber	protein
DAILY TOTALS					

ENERGY LEVEL

1 2 3 4 5 6 7 8 9 10

LOW ——— HIGH

STRESS LEVEL

1 2 3 4 5 6 7 8 9 10

LOW ——— HIGH

EXERCISE

time	type	duration

NOTES

DAY FIVE

date: ______________ S M T W T F S sleep hours: ________

fasting blood sugar: ______________ time: __________ am pm

MORNING

blood sugar: __________ time: __________ am pm

food/drink	calories	fat	carbs	fiber	protein
totals:					

medication: ______________________ dose: __________ time: __________ am pm

post-meal blood sugar: __________ time: __________ am pm

SNACK

blood sugar: __________ time: __________ am pm

food/drink	calories	fat	carbs	fiber	protein

medication: ______________________ dose: __________ time: __________ am pm

post-meal blood sugar: __________ time: __________ am pm

MIDDAY

blood sugar: __________ time: __________ am pm

food/drink	calories	fat	carbs	fiber	protein
totals:					

medication: ______________________ dose: __________ time: __________ am pm

post-meal blood sugar: __________ time: __________ am pm

SNACK

blood sugar: __________ time: __________ am pm

food/drink	calories	fat	carbs	fiber	protein

medication: ______________________ dose: __________ time: __________ am pm

post-meal blood sugar: __________ time: __________ am pm

EVENING blood sugar: ____________ time: ____________ am pm

food/drink	calories	fat	carbs	fiber	protein
totals:					

medication: ____________ dose: ____________ time: ____________ am pm

post-meal blood sugar: ____________ time: ____________ am pm

NIGHT blood sugar: ____________ time: ____________ am pm

food/drink	calories	fat	carbs	fiber	protein

medication: ____________ dose: ____________ time: ____________ am pm

post-meal blood sugar: ____________ time: ____________ am pm

AVG B.S.	

	calories	fat	carbs	fiber	protein
DAILY TOTALS					

ENERGY LEVEL

1 2 3 4 5 6 7 8 9 10

LOW —— HIGH

STRESS LEVEL

1 2 3 4 5 6 7 8 9 10

LOW —— HIGH

EXERCISE

time	type	duration

NOTES

DAY SIX

date: ____________ S M T W T F S sleep hours: ____________

fasting blood sugar: ____________ time: ____________ am pm

MORNING blood sugar: ____________ time: ____________ am pm

food/drink	calories	fat	carbs	fiber	protein
totals:					

medication: ____________ dose: ____________ time: ____________ am pm

post-meal blood sugar: ____________ time: ____________ am pm

SNACK blood sugar: ____________ time: ____________ am pm

food/drink	calories	fat	carbs	fiber	protein

medication: ____________ dose: ____________ time: ____________ am pm

post-meal blood sugar: ____________ time: ____________ am pm

MIDDAY blood sugar: ____________ time: ____________ am pm

food/drink	calories	fat	carbs	fiber	protein
totals:					

medication: ____________ dose: ____________ time: ____________ am pm

post-meal blood sugar: ____________ time: ____________ am pm

SNACK blood sugar: ____________ time: ____________ am pm

food/drink	calories	fat	carbs	fiber	protein

medication: ____________ dose: ____________ time: ____________ am pm

post-meal blood sugar: ____________ time: ____________ am pm

EVENING blood sugar: ____________ time: ____________ am pm

food/drink	calories	fat	carbs	fiber	protein
totals:					

medication: __________________________ dose: __________ time: ________ am pm

post-meal blood sugar: ____________ time: ____________ am pm

NIGHT blood sugar: ____________ time: ____________ am pm

food/drink	calories	fat	carbs	fiber	protein

medication: __________________________ dose: __________ time: ________ am pm

post-meal blood sugar: ____________ time: ____________ am pm

AVG B.S.	

	calories	fat	carbs	fiber	protein
DAILY TOTALS					

ENERGY LEVEL

1 2 3 4 5 6 7 8 9 10

LOW ———————— HIGH

STRESS LEVEL

1 2 3 4 5 6 7 8 9 10

LOW ———————— HIGH

EXERCISE

time	type	duration

NOTES

DAY SEVEN

date: ____________ S M T W T F S sleep hours: ________

fasting blood sugar: ____________ time: ________ am pm

MORNING blood sugar: ________ time: ________ am pm

food/drink	calories	fat	carbs	fiber	protein
totals:					

medication: ____________ dose: ________ time: ________ am pm

post-meal blood sugar: ________ time: ________ am pm

SNACK blood sugar: ________ time: ________ am pm

food/drink	calories	fat	carbs	fiber	protein

medication: ____________ dose: ________ time: ________ am pm

post-meal blood sugar: ________ time: ________ am pm

MIDDAY blood sugar: ________ time: ________ am pm

food/drink	calories	fat	carbs	fiber	protein
totals:					

medication: ____________ dose: ________ time: ________ am pm

post-meal blood sugar: ________ time: ________ am pm

SNACK blood sugar: ________ time: ________ am pm

food/drink	calories	fat	carbs	fiber	protein

medication: ____________ dose: ________ time: ________ am pm

post-meal blood sugar: ________ time: ________ am pm

EVENING blood sugar: ________ time: ________ am pm

food/drink	calories	fat	carbs	fiber	protein
totals:					

medication: ________ dose: ________ time: ________ am pm

post-meal blood sugar: ________ time: ________ am pm

NIGHT blood sugar: ________ time: ________ am pm

food/drink	calories	fat	carbs	fiber	protein

medication: ________ dose: ________ time: ________ am pm

post-meal blood sugar: ________ time: ________ am pm

AVG B.S.	

	calories	fat	carbs	fiber	protein
DAILY TOTALS					

ENERGY LEVEL

1 2 3 4 5 6 7 8 9 10

LOW —— HIGH

STRESS LEVEL

1 2 3 4 5 6 7 8 9 10

LOW —— HIGH

EXERCISE

time	type	duration

NOTES

WEEK SIX

WEEKLY SUMMARY

BLOOD SUGAR

day	MORNING pre	MORNING post	SNACK pre	SNACK post	MIDDAY pre	MIDDAY post	SNACK pre	SNACK post	EVENING pre	EVENING post	NIGHT pre	NIGHT post
1												
2												
3												
4												
5												
6												
7												
AVG.												

MACROS

day	calories	fat	carbs	fiber	protein
1					
2					
3					
4					
5					
6					
7					
AVG.					

NOTES

ENERGY LEVEL AVERAGE

1 2 3 4 5 6 7 8 9 10

LOW —— HIGH

STRESS LEVEL AVERAGE

1 2 3 4 5 6 7 8 9 10

LOW —— HIGH

DAYS OF EXERCISE

1 2 3 4 5 6 7

AVG. MIN.

____

GOALS MET

ADJUSTMENTS

NOTES

Things I learned over the last six weeks:

-
-
-
-
-

Things to talk about with my doctor:

-
-
-
-
-

Other notes:

-
-

NOTES

NOTES

NOTES

NOTES

BONUS MATERIAL

MEAL PLANNER TEMPLATE

Download 6 free meal planning templates to choose from, and get 10 helpful meal planning tips.

https://devotionsondiabetes.com/diabetes-meal-plan-made-easy/

DIABETIC FOOD LIST AND GROCERY LIST

Download a list of the best foods for diabetics and also a grocery list template to print and use.

https://devotionsondiabetes.com/quick-and-easy-breakfast-ideas-for-type-1-diabetes/

HABIT TRACKER PRINTABLES

Track literally any habit you'd like with these free monthly habit tracker printables.

https://devotionsondiabetes.com/the-habits-we-keep-and-a-new-circle-habit-tracker-printable/

For many more free downloads on various diabetes-related topics, visit www.DevotionsOnDiabetes.com.

DID YOU ENJOY THIS BOOK?

Thank you for using this blood sugar log book. Would you consider sharing this with someone else?

Here are a few ideas:

- Write a review where you purchased this book.

- Post about it on social media using #DevotionsOnDiabetes.

- Purchase a copy for a friend or family member.

- Sign up for weekly blog emails at DevotionsOnDiabetes.com.

- Connect with us online:
  Blog website: DevotionsOnDiabetes.com
  Facebook: Devotions On Diabetes
  Instagram: @DevotionsOnDiabetes

Thank you in advance!

ABOUT THE CREATOR

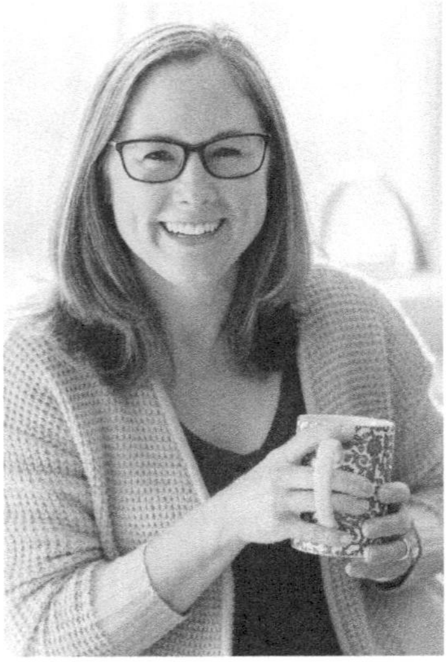

Diagnosed at age 12, Kaycee has lived with type 1 diabetes for more than 30 years.

With her degree in journalism and a storyteller's heart, she has been writing books and blog posts about diabetes for several years. She loves to share about the connection between faith and illness, life with diabetes, and diabetic-friendly food. You can find her work at DevotionsOnDiabetes.com.

Kaycee and her husband have a love for God's Word and discipleship, two beautiful children, and a rapidly aging dog. She enjoys treating highs with insulin, treating lows with marshmallow fluff straight from the spoon, and treating diabetes as an opportunity to seek God and point others to Him.

Kaycee is also the author of *Devotions on Diabetes: A 30-Day Journey to Anchor Your Soul*, available on Amazon.

devotionsondiabetes.com

MORE FROM THE AUTHOR

Devotions on Diabetes: A 30-Day Journey to Anchor Your Soul

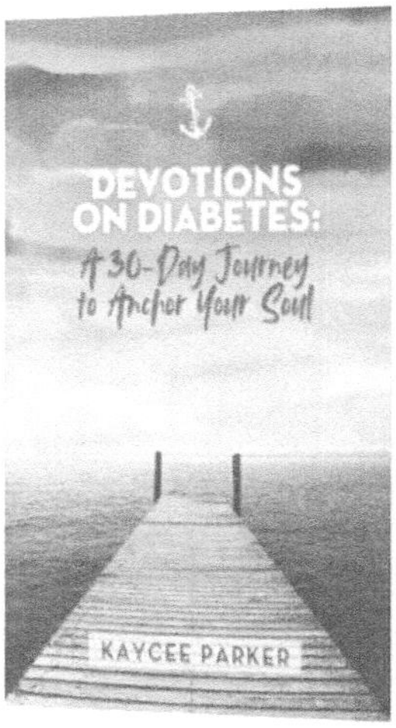

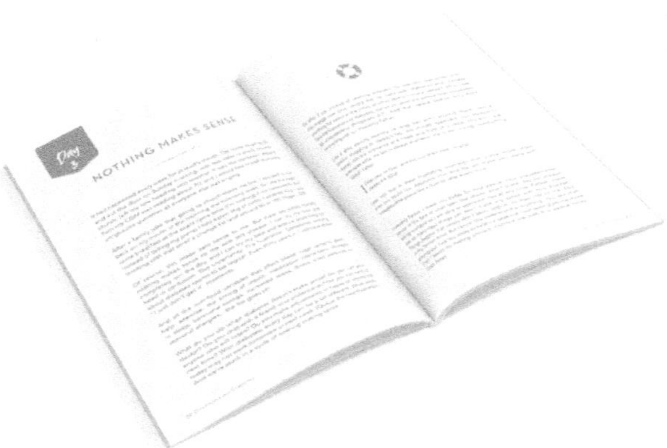

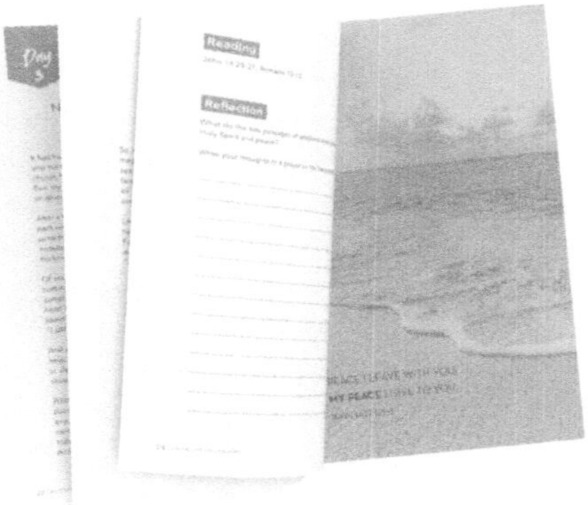

Life with diabetes can be unpredictable. It can feel overwhelming, complicated, and exhausting. But we can be secure and grounded through it all.

You are invited on a 30-day journey to discover how this is possible. Are you ready to anchor your soul?

Complete with 30 days of devotions, this book also includes:

- personal stories
- biblical application
- reflection questions
- additional suggested readings
- room for notes and prayers

This book was written to relate to and encourage anyone who deals with diabetes, and to view it all through the lens of the Bible.

Purchase on Amazon

Made in the USA
Middletown, DE
05 November 2026

36560129R00066